ROSACEA: I CURED MY ROSACEA IN TWO DAYS! YOU CAN TOO!

By R. Kelly Jones RDN,M.A.,M.Msc

Copyright 2015

TABLE OF CONTENTS

Living With Rosacea

CHAPTER 1

INTRODUCTION

Congratulations, you have taken the first step in curing your rosacea. I cured my rosacea in **TWO DAYS** and have not had a flare up of rosacea for ten years. You are about to learn the inexpensive topical treatment that cured my rosacea in just **TWO DAYS!** You will learn the proper cleansers, toners, and moisturizers to use to keep your skin looking flawless. You will learn the supplements that are beneficial to your complexion and the supplements that can aggravate rosacea. You will learn how to soothe the burn of rosacea instantly. You will learn the safest hair coloring, shampoos and cosmetics to use.

I had been a rosacea sufferer for over twenty years, when I rubbed a common substance on my face and in two days my rosacea was gone. I have not had a flare up of my rosacea in years and I consider my rosacea cured. I have spent thousands of dollars and conducted hundreds of hours of research trying to control my rosacea. There are many expensive supplements and facial products that say they are specifically formulated for rosacea sufferers. In the past, I tried many of these and they did not control my rosacea. I still had flare ups. I have gotten amazing results from the inexpensive products and easy protocol you will be reading about in this book. I want to save you money and time. More importantly, I want to help you regain your self-confidence by having the best complexion that you can. My complexion has never looked better!

It all started one day when I looked in the mirror and saw a red blotch on my left cheek approximately two inches in diameter. The red blotch came and went. I began my search to find out what was going on by going to my family physician. My family physician did not know what I had and I saw five dermatologists in eight years before being properly diagnosed.

During this time, I became aware of foods, certain weather conditions and activities that caused my face to become red and burn. I began to avoid these triggers that included salad dressing, hot beverages, tomato sauce, spicy food, wind, exercise, sun and cold weather. I also found that most sunscreens caused my face to turn red. I started wearing a large brimmed hat in the summer because both the sun and sunscreen caused a worsening of my symptoms.

Being diagnosed with rosacea is difficult emotionally and physically. Rosacea does hurt physically. Often my face burned so bad that I could not sleep. I watched my pretty complexion that brought me compliments, replaced by red blotchy skin.

I also discovered that I had ocular rosacea, which caused my eyes to look red and itch. I began to lose my eyelashes and eyebrows and again I saw several ophthalmologists before I was correctly diagnosed with ocular rosacea. There is more awareness of rosacea than ever before, so diagnosis should not be difficult. I do recommend seeing a physician for diagnosis.

CHAPTER 2

SYMPTOMS, CAUSES AND MEDICAL TREATMENTS OF ROSACEA:

Rosacea is a common skin condition characterized by transient or persistent facial redness, visible blood vessels often with papules and pustules and a burning sensation of the face. Redness of the face may occur only on the cheeks or include the forehead, chin, and nose. You can have rosacea on your scalp, neck, ears and chest. There are four broad categories of rosacea: 1.Erythematotelangectatic, which is the redness, stinging and burning of rosacea. 2. Papulopustular, which is the raised discolored skin of rosacea. Papules are the raised discolored bubbles of the skin that are solid without visible fluid. Pustules are similar to papules but are instead filled with pus. 3. Phymatous, this is the stage of rosacea where thickening of the skin, enlargement or irregular surface nodularities occur. 4. Ocular rosacea which causes red, itchy, burning eyes with swollen eyelids. You may feel like you have sand in your eyes. Ocular rosacea can lead to eyelash loss. Rosacea can also cause itching and loss of eyebrows.

The cause of rosacea is still unknown. Hypotheses include vascular abnormalities, dermal matrix degeneration, environmental factors and microorganisms such as Dermodex folliculorum and Helicobacter pylori. The most recent medical research has found that rosacea sufferers have a higher amount of a protein called Toll-like receptor 2 (TLR2) as part of their immune system. This may cause an increased inflammatory response to environmental stimuli.

While there are medical treatments aimed at controlling the symptoms of rosacea, these treatments do not cure rosacea. Topical prescription medical treatments for facial rosacea include metronidazole, azelaic acid, sulfur and retinoids. Oral medications include the antibiotics metronidazole, tetracyclines and macrolides. The antibiotic docycycline is the oral antibiotic most often used to treat ocular rosacea.

Chapter 3

Common Triggers of Rosacea:

1. Spicy foods, including garlic, pepper, salsa, salad dressing and msg.

2. Hot weather.

3. Cold weather.

4. Wind.

5. Sun.

6. Hot beverages like coffee and tea.

7. Physical exertion.

8. Certain cosmetics.

9. Some sunscreens.

10. Some moisturizers.

11. Hot bath, shower, sauna.

12. Stress.

13. Menopause (Hot Flashes).

14. Alcohol.

You may also discover triggers that are unique to you. It may be helpful to keep a log to discover your personal triggers and avoid these until your rosacea is better.

How I Cured My Rosacea:

CHAPTER 4

CLEANSING YOUR FACE:

I wash my face in the morning and before going to bed. I use cool to lukewarm water and I use only my hands. I go over my entire face, moving my hands in a circular motion. I rinse my face well, splashing my face eight to twelve times with water. I gently pat my face dry with a soft towel. If your face is dry you can skip the cleanser in the morning and just rinse your face with cool water.

You can start with the following cleansers:

Product:	Where to Find Product:
Unscented Dove bar soap	Local grocery store or Amazon.com
Oil of Olay Cleansing Facial Foam for sensitive skin.	Amazon.com
Keys Island Rx Therapeutic Foaming Facial Cleanser	Amazon.com
The Body Shop Aloe Calming Facial Cleanser	Amazon.com
Thayer's alcohol-free original witch hazel with aloe vera	Amazon.com
T.N. Dickinson's witch hazel	Amazon.com

I use Thayer's or Dickinson's witch hazel as a toner. I recommend using Thayer's alcohol-free original witch hazel with aloe vera to begin with. I do fine with Dickinson's witch hazel. It does contain a small amount of alcohol which may irritate some people. After washing with unscented Dove soap and drying my face, I put the witch hazel on a cotton ball and wipe my entire face and neck. This deep cleans without aggravating rosacea.

Chapter 5

Beneficial Topical Treatments. The Topical Treatment That Cured My Rosacea.

Product:	Where to Find Product:
Apple Cider Vinegar (I prefer organic)	Amazon.com
Vitamin K serum or cream	Amazon.com
Critical Care Calming Gel	Amazon.com
Aubrey Organics Pure Aloe Vera	Amazon.com
LaRoche-Posey Thermal Spring Water	Amazon.com
Dermalogica Ultracalming Mist	www.greatskin.com
CV Skinlabs Rescue & Relief Spray	www.cvskinlabs.com
Metronidazole Cream	Physician prescription

I have listed the treatment products in order of impact on clearing my rosacea. After washing your face and using the witch hazel, gently put the apple cider vinegar solution over your entire face using a cotton ball. Make the apple cider vinegar solution by mixing 1 part apple cider vinegar with 2 parts water. For example, when making a cup of this solution use 2/3 cup of water mixed with 1/3 cup of apple cider vinegar. If you don't want to store the mixture, you can mix

2 tablespoons of water with 1 tablespoon of apple cider vinegar every time you want to use the solution. I started using the apple cider vinegar solution twice a day, morning and evening, and in two days my face was glowing. I had no signs of rosacea and my pores appeared smaller. I have not had a flare up of rosacea since that day. I highly recommend starting your treatment of rosacea using apple cider vinegar. Once my face was clear I reduced the use of the apple cider vinegar and presently use it no more than once a week, and sometimes go months without using it.

Vitamin K serum strengthens the blood vessels and it is **very effective** in controlling the redness of rosacea. Claudia Stevens is the brand that I found to be the most effective, unfortunately it is no longer available. There are several brands of vitamin K serums and creams available at Amazon.com. I personally found vitamin K serum to be more effective in reducing redness than vitamin K cream. I currently am not using a vitamin K serum because I don't need to.

The Critical Care Calming Gel can be applied after the apple cider vinegar has dried and the name says it all. If your face is red and burning the Critical Care Calming Gel will immediately have a soothing effect on your face. You can use this twice a day as well. You don't need a lot so be careful squeezing the tube as it comes out quickly. This product does contain small amounts of parabens and propylene glycol. I still recommend using this product for rosacea that burns and is sore. I found a small amount was all I needed to use and it did help me. I have not needed to use it in years. I believe it can be a beneficial product in the short term until your rosacea is better. If you want to avoid parabens and propylene glycol, try Aubrey Organics Pure Aloe Vera. When I was using this product I kept it in my refrigerator and used it as a moisturizer. The cool gel felt great and it soothed my skin.

The LaRoche-Posey Thermal Spring Water also calms a burning face. This is great to keep close by to spray on your face after exercise or anytime your face burns. It also contains minerals including zinc, selenium and magnesium to nourish your skin and protect against free radicals. I also like the Dermalogica Ultracalming Mist and the CV Skinlabs Rescue & Relief Spray. The LaRoche-Posey spray and Ultracalming Mist are both fragrance free. The CV Skinlabs Rescue & Relief Spray has a light cucumber scent. I personally prefer fragrance free products.

While I did find the prescription Metronidazole Cream effective in controlling some of my rosacea symptoms, I still had to be diligent in avoiding all of my triggers. I stopped using metronidazole cream years ago.

If you are struggling with broken capillaries on your face you may want to consider a photofacial procedure. This is done at a dermatologist's office, using intense pulsed light. You will be given a pair of dark glasses to wear. The procedure feels a little like a hot elastic hitting your face. It is a very tolerable procedure. This procedure will irritate your skin a little but in a few days to a week your skin will look better.

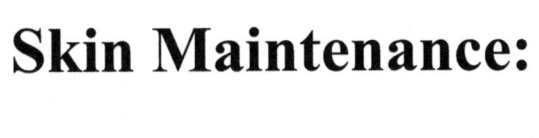

Skin Maintenance:

CHAPTER 6

SUNSCREEN:

I recommend that you wear sunscreen every day. The brands that I like best are:

Product:	Where to Find Product:
TI-SILC SHEER	Amazon.com
Solar Rx	Amazon.com
Honest sunscreen	Honestcompany.com

My favorite sunscreen is the Honest brand in the squeeze tube because it contains non-nano zinc oxide which has healing properties.

CHAPTER 7

MOISTURIZERS:

I avoid heavy moisturizers especially when going to bed. I find heavy moisturizers can aggravate rosacea at night. The following are light moisturizers that I have been able to use successfully.

Product:	Where to Find Product:
Aubrey Organics Pure Aloe Vera Gel	Amazon.com
Rhonda Allison Moisture Au Lait	www.greatskin.com
Visual Changes Lactic Nutrient Crème	www.kimberlyspa.com
Note: Visual Changes does contain parabens.	
Pure hyaluronic acid serum	Amazon.com
Livpurely coconut cream	Amazon.com
Argan oil	Vitacost.com

Rhonda Allison's Moisture Au Lait is a wonderful moisturizer and will make your skin look amazing. It does contain a small amount of retinol, which potentially could cause irritation in some. The small amount of retinol in Rhonda Allison's Moisture Au Lait very gently exfoliates the skin and I've found Moisture Au Lait to be a great moisturizer making my skin look flawless. I personally don't recommend using prescription strength retinol on rosacea. The Moisture Au Lait has the perfect amount of retinol to gently exfoliate the skin. If you want to wait until your rosacea is better before using this moisturizer you can use the Aubrey Organics Pure Aloe Vera Gel.

While I was using Visual Changes Lactic Nutrient Crème I found it helped reduce redness and improved my complexion. It contains lactic acid which is good for rosacea. The Visual Changes moisturizer does contain parabens and I have decided to stop using products containing parabens, propylene glycol, sodium hydroxide(lye) and phthalates. Parabens and phthalates may promote certain cancers and propylene glycol is a known irritant to skin, although when I have used products containing propylene glycol I have had no problem. I also recommend avoiding the ingredient dimethicone (until your rosacea is better) commonly found in moisturizers and foundations. Although dimethicone is generally considered safe, it coats your skin and can clog pores and aggravate rosacea.

The Livpurely coconut cream moisturizer has a greasier feel and is heavier than the other moisturizers. It's great when your face is feeling dry. I use this moisturizer occasionally during the day when my face is feeling dry. I have tried many brands of hyaluronic acid serum and none of them have irritated my skin.

I have used several argan oil brands and have done well with all of them. I am currently using glonaturals brand of argan oil available from vitacost.com. Argan oil does have the consistency of oil. You can use it sparingly on wrinkles. I like it because I use it on my hair and nails and it makes my hair and nails shine.

Chapter 8

Cosmetics:

It is important to use cosmetics that do not irritate your skin. The following is a list of cosmetics that I use successfully. They are paraben, phthalate and fragrance free and do no animal testing.

Product:	Where to Find Product:
Jill Iredale products	Amazon.com
Coastal Classic Creations	www.coastalclassiccreations.com
It Cosmetics	Amazon.com
Real Purity	Amazon.com
Dr. Hauschka	Amazon.com
Laura Geller	Amazon.com
Lorac cosmetics	Amazon.com
Ecco Bella	www.eccobella.com

I have been using It Cosmetic's eyebrow pencil, which facilitates hair growth, and I have experienced less itching in my eyebrow area. I have also been using their eyeliner without increased itching. Jill Iredale has a good eyeliner as well.

There are green tinted moisturizers that can be worn under your foundation to counteract the redness of rosacea if needed, until your rosacea is better. Dermalogica Ultracalming Redness Relief is one that I like and it has a SPF of 20. This can be purchased at www.greatskin.com. I have not needed to use this in years.

Jill Iredale's BB cream and liquid mineral foundation are wonderful and they make your complexion look amazing. I am currently using Real Purity's foundation and lipstick. The foundation has only six ingredients and gives a beautiful medium coverage. The lipsticks are beautiful and they provide samples so you can pick the best shade for your skin tone.

I am currently using Lorac double feature concealer/highlighter and I find it easy to apply. It happens to be my favorite under eye concealer.

Dr. Hauschka's products do not contain paraben or chemical fragrances. Some of the products do contain essential oils that add a fragrance.

CHAPTER 9

BROWN SPOTS:

If you have hyper-pigmented areas on your face that you want to fade, I recommend meladerm available at Amazon.com. This product is free from hydroquinone. It works slowly and is gentle on your skin. The Moisture Au Lait will help reduce hyper-pigmented areas as well.

Chapter 10

Supplements:

Always consult your physician before starting a supplement program. Some rosacea suffers see improvement in their symptoms while taking a L-Lysine supplement. L-Lysine is an amino acid naturally found in high protein foods like eggs, and meat. Some feel that a deficiency of L-Lysine is causing their rosacea. I tried a L-Lysine supplement at 1000-2000mg. daily and this had a slight effect on reducing my rosacea symptoms but not a significant effect. L-Lysine supplements can be found at your local pharmacy or at Amazon.com.

Some rosacea sufferers report benefit from taking betaine HCL a hydrochloric acid supplement with the premise that low levels of hydrochloric acid in the stomach is causing their rosacea. Signs of low hydrochloric acid levels are acid reflux, heartburn, burping, gas, bloating or nausea after eating. If you have any of these symptoms I recommend talking with your physician before taking hydrochloric acid supplements. Taking large doses of hydrochloric acid supplements can burn the stomach lining.

Omega-3 fatty acids can improve the condition of your skin. Take according to the instructions on the omega-3 supplement label. Some brands that I trust are OmegaBrite, Seroyal Super EFA Capsules and Terry Naturally Vectomega. All of these can be ordered at Amazon.com. If you are taking anti-coagulants, medicines to thin your blood, consult your physician before starting an omega-3 fatty acid supplement.

If you are taking a multivitamin or vitamin B supplement check to see how much vitamin B 12 is present. Consumerlab.com reports that doses of 20mcg or more of vitamin B 12 daily may contribute to acne and rosacea.

From my personal experience, I found that ascorbic acid (vitamin C) supplements can aggravate rosacea. The ascorbate form of vitamin C did not aggravate my rosacea. Vitamin C is good for our skin so try to eat foods high in vitamin C every day. Foods high in vitamin C include: red and green peppers, oranges, grapefruit, kiwi, tomato, brussels sprouts, strawberries, cantaloupe, broccoli, kale, spinach, guava, acerola cherries, papayas, and cauliflower. If you want to continue to take a vitamin C supplement I would recommend the ascorbate form (ascorbate will be listed on the label) at no higher than 200mg. per day to start.

CHAPTER 11

PILLOWCASES:

Yes, pillowcases can make a difference. I recommend buying satin at a fabric shop and making your own pillow cases. You can buy satin pillowcases in stores but they are not always easy to find. The satin is gentle on red inflamed skin. Be sure to get enough sleep (8-9 hours every night) so your skin can heal.

Chapter 12

Hair Coloring:

I recommend pure natural ingredients for coloring your hair. Hair dyes contain chemicals that can cause allergies and scalp irritations. Even many of the hair coloring kits, including henna coloring kits, found in health food stores contain chemicals. I use pure henna and Dutch cocoa to color my hair. Body art quality henna can be purchased at Butters-N-Bars.com or Mehandi.com. An added benefit is that body art quality henna can calm an itchy scalp. I find the staff at both Butters-N-Bars.com and Mehandi.com to be knowledgeable and very helpful. I highly recommend both of these sites. Although pure henna can only dye your hair red, indigo can be added to give varying shades of brown and there are natural products that can give hair a blonde tint. The staff at both of these sites can help you decide what you need for the color result you want.

CHAPTER 13

TAKE CARE OF YOUR SCALP:

Pay attention to your scalp. Does it itch? Is it flakey? If so, get these symptoms under control. Scalp conditions occur at a higher rate in people with facial rosacea than in people without rosacea. T-gel shampoo, a tar based shampoo, can be helpful in controlling an itchy scalp. For particularly stubborn itch, use maximum strength scalpicin in the 1.5 fl. oz. bottle. It contains 1% hydrocortisone. Use according to directions on the label. Scalpicin can be used on your eyebrows if you are experiencing itching in this area. Put a drop of scalpicin on a Q tip and wipe over your eyebrow area. This can be used short term to get the itching under control if needed. You can wipe the apple cider vinegar solution over your eyebrow area as well. Do not use scalpicin, or any other over the counter steroid, on your lash line. Do not get scalpicin in your eyes.

For a more natural approach to treating an itchy scalp, Just Natural Scalp shampoo can be tried. I currently don't need to use an anti itch shampoo. I am using Aubrey's Blue Chamomile shampoo and Stonybrook Botanicals unscented Herbal Oil-free shampoo. They are both paraben and phthalate free. Another great option is a shampoo and body wash called Everyday Shea Butter Shampoo & Body Wash, Calming Lemon-Lavender. This shampoo scored a 10, the highest safety score possible, from GoodGuide.com. All of these shampoos can be ordered online at Amazon.com.

I use Real Purity's "Hair Spray Sensitive." It's a light hair spray and works well. Remember what you spray on your hair, you spray on your face. Available at Amazon.com.

CHAPTER 14

NATURAL PRODUCTS:

I personally believe in the use of as few chemicals as possible on our skin and hair. The Environmental Working Group is a valuable resource in helping you determine the safety of the products you are using. Here is the address for their website: www.ewg.org.

CHAPTER 15

NUTRITION AND EXERCISE:

B eing a registered dietitian, I believe good nutrition and proper exercise is important for everyone. Eating foods high in nutritional value will provide the nutrients needed for healthy skin. Try these basic nutrition tips. 1. Eat at least five servings of a combination of fruits and vegetables every day. One serving is equal to one cup of raw or one-half cup of cooked vegetables, or one medium size fresh fruit such as an apple. It is best to eat a variety of fruits and vegetables. Buy organic when you can. 2. Eat whole grains; when buying cereals and breads look for the word whole grain on the label. 3. Eat lean sources of protein, these include lean cuts of meat, beans, and low fat cheeses. Salmon and sardines are good sources of protein and omega 3 fatty acids. They have natural anti-inflammatory properties so they are beneficial to the health of our skin. I recommend eating wild caught salmon or wild caught sardines (because they are low in mercury) one to two times per week. Flaxseeds (buy ground flaxseeds or grind them yourself so you can absorb the omega 3 fatty acids) and walnuts are also great sources of omega-3 fatty acids. 4. Avoid eating fried and processed foods on a regular basis. 5. Avoid foods and beverages high in sugar including soda and fruit juices as these can cause inflammation and aggravate rosacea. 6. Avoid foods high in sodium (salt) like pickles, salted crackers, pretzels, chips, and lunch meat. These foods can cause fluid retention and also cause the inflammation of rosacea to be worse. 7. Drink water throughout the day. In general, most adults need 6-8 glasses of water a day. 9. For some people dairy and wheat can cause inflammation. 10. Avoid alcohol completely. 11. Avoid spicy food such as chili, tacos, burritos, lasagna, hot peppers, BBQ chips. 12. Avoid foods containing hot spices like taco seasoning, salad dressings, tomato/spaghetti sauce, tabasco sauce, salsa, BBQ sauce, onion powder, garlic, black pepper, red pepper flakes, baharat seasoning, cayenne pepper, curry powder, chili powder, aleppo pepper, cajun sauce, ginger. 13. Avoid hot beverages like tea and coffee.

Once your rosacea is better you can gradually add back some of the restricted foods to your diet. It use to be necessary for me to avoid a wide variety of foods. Currently no food makes my rosacea flare. I don't like extremely spicy food so I don't eat things like tabasco sauce or pepper. I am able to eat the foods that I like including tacos, spaghetti sauce and salad dressings without having a flare up of rosacea.

Exercise is important in reducing stress levels to help control your rosacea. Yoga and meditation are also helpful in reducing stress levels and will help get your rosacea under control. Some of you will experience a flare up of your rosacea with vigorous exercise. If you do, try walking at a leisurely pace. You can also carry a spray bottle filled with cool water with you to spray your face to keep it cool during exercise. You can also use the LaRoche-Posey Thermal Spring Water to spray your face. You won't need this once your rosacea is better.

CHAPTER 16

SUMMARY:

Because I no longer experience flare ups of my rosacea, my current cleansing, moisturizing and makeup routine includes; washing my face with Dove soap am and pm followed by witch hazel in the pm, Rhonda Allison Moisture Au Lait, hyaluronic acid serum, argan oil or Livpurely Coconut Moisturizer. I rotate the moisturizers. I use Honest sunscreen daily in the am. I continue to use Jill Iredale, Real Purity, Lorac, Dr. Hauschka, Laura Geller and It cosmetics. Because my skin no longer reacts to triggers I only use the vinegar solution occasionally because it makes my pores look smaller, but I no longer need it to control my rosacea. The frequency of use of the vinegar solution will vary individually based on your needs.

Topical Rosacea Treatment Routine:

Morning Routine:

*Wash your face with a mild cleanser, unscented Dove soap is fine. Rinse with cool water. Pat dry. If your face is very dry, just rinse it with cool water and skip washing it with Dove soap until your skin's condition has improved.

*Apply the vinegar solution morning and night until your face is better, then you can try reducing the use of it.

*Apply Vitamin K serum (optional).

*If you are using the prescription metronidazole cream and want to continue using it you can apply it after the vinegar solution or vitamin K serum has dried.

*If your face is burning, apply the Critical Care Calming Gel or Aubrey-Organics Pure Aloe Vera Gel after the vinegar solution has dried or after the vitamin K serum has dried or after applying the metronidazole cream if you are using either of these products.

*Spray your face with LaRoche-Posey Thermal Spring water, Dermalogica Ultracalming Spray or the Rescue & Relief Spray (optional).

*Apply a small amount of the Rhonda Allison Moisture Au Lait. Once your rosacea is better you can start to use the other moisturizers mentioned in this book.

*Apply sunscreen.

*Apply your cosmetics if you choose to use makeup.

Evening Routine:

*Wash your face with a mild cleanser, unscented Dove soap is fine. Rinse with cool water. Pat dry.

*Apply alcohol free witch hazel. I like to use the witch hazel in the evening because it deep cleans the grime of the day.

*Apply the vinegar solution.

*Apply Vitamin K serum (optional).

*If you are using the prescription metronidazole cream you can apply it after the vinegar solution or Vitamin K serum has dried.

*If your face is burning, apply the Critical Care Calming Gel or Aubrey-Organics Pure Aloe Vera Gel after the vinegar solution or Vitamin K serum has dried or after applying the metronidazole cream if you are using either of these products.

*Spray your face with LaRoche-Posey Thermal Spring water, Dermalogica Ultracalming Spray or the Rescue & Relief Spray (optional).

*Apply a small amount of the Rhonda Allison Moisture Au Lait. You may want to avoid moisturizes at night until your rosacea is better. When you do start using a moisturizer as part of your evening routine, be sure the moisturizer has completely dried before going to bed.

You will be able to streamline your topical treatment once your rosacea is better.

Recap:

If you are feeling overwhelmed remember:

Once your rosacea symptoms are gone, your maintenance routine will be: wash with unscented Dove soap, tone with witch hazel, use apple cider vinegar as needed and moisturize with Moisture Au Lait and your skin will look fantastic!

It really is that simple. You can use the other products mentioned in this book as needed and or as you want.

Curing my rosacea has saved me hundreds of dollars and I no longer have to live my life in fear of my rosacea flaring up. I am now able to eat salad dressing, spaghetti sauce and burritos, exercise vigorously, enjoy being outside on a sunny, windy day and drink a cup of hot chocolate without symptoms of rosacea flaring. I am confident that you will be able do to these things again too! There is nothing I have to avoid because of rosacea. My rosacea is a thing of the past!

Follow the protocol outlined in this book and your rosacea will be a thing of the past very soon!

CHAPTER 17

HOW TO RELIEVE THE SYMPTOMS OF OCULAR ROSACEA

About 60% of people with facial rosacea develop ocular rosacea. Symptoms of ocular rosacea include; dry eyes, sties, tearing, burning, red, itchy eyes, and loss of eye lashes. You may feel like you have sand or grit in your eyes. Your eyes may be sensitive to light and you may have red swollen eye lids. I wear sunglasses when I drive and when I am outside. You can also experience itching and loss of your eyelashes. Ocular rosacea can be serious if the cornea is involved. I recommend seeing a physician for proper diagnosis. Continue to have regular eye exams.

A warm washcloth placed on the eyes will help soothe them and will help distribute the oils in blocked eyelid glands helping to lubricate the eye. Try doing this for five minutes morning and evening. If placing a warm washcloth on your eyes aggravates your facial rosacea, use cool water on your washcloth until your facial rosacea is better, then you can use a warm washcloth. This simple act will help a lot.

You will need to wash your eyelids with an eyelid scrub. I like OcuSoft Foaming Eyelid Cleanser, available at Amazon.com. Wash your hands first, then squirt a small amount of cleanser on your index finger. With your eyes closed, gently rub the cleanser across your lid on the lash line for about 15 seconds. Do this morning and evening. Please do this gently, vigorous rubbing could cause your eyelashes to fall out. This will not sting your eyes. During a flare up you can use OcuSoft *plus* Foaming Eyelid Cleanser. This will sting if you get it in your eyes, so be sure to keep your eyes closed.

If you have allergies, you may be experiencing itching caused from your allergies as well as from your rosacea. I am currently using Zaditor eye drops, available at Amazon. com or your local pharmacy and it works as well as prescription strength anti itch eye drops. You are going to need to use artificial tears liberally, four to eight times a day. There are several available, experiment to see which one works best for you. I am currently using Systane and Thera Tears. Both are available at Amazon.com or your local pharmacy.

If you have very dry eyes you may need the prescription eye drop Restasis. Restasis reduces inflammation and helps improve tear production. This has been beneficial for me. The prescription eye drop Alrex is a steroid so it needs to be used with caution because it can increase ocular pressure. I have found this very helpful if I am experiencing excessive eyelash lost. I don't put the drop in my eye. I put a drop on my index finger, after washing my hands, and then I gently rub the Alrex drop on the base of my eyelashes. This will help reduce inflammation and reduce eyelash loss. Do not use an over the counter steroid, like scalpicin, in your eyes. Using an eye lid scrub, Restasis, Alrex, Zaditor and artificial tears eye drops has been beneficial for me in keeping my eyelashes healthy and preventing breakage and loss.

Eyebrows and eyelashes can be very slow to grow back once they are lost. I have tried many products and have found a product called Talika eyelash conditioning cream to work the best in accelerating the growth of both my eyelashes and eyebrows. This can be purchased online at Amazon.com.

Be sure to use cosmetics that do not aggravate your ocular rosacea. I use Jane Iredale and It cosmetics eyeliner. I don't use mascara. If you want to try mascara I recommend Jane Iredale's mascara for sensitive eyes. You can also use Talika lipocils eyelash conditioning gel. It is a clear gel that you apply like mascara and it will prevent your lashes from becoming dry and brittle.

Follow the protocol in this book and say good-bye to your ocular rosacea symptoms.

References:

- Crawford, G., Pelle, M., James, W., Rosacea: I. Etiology, pathogenesis, and subtype classification. Journal of the American Academy of Dermatology, vol. 51, issue 3, September 2004, pages 327-341.

- Parodi, A., Drago, S., Paolino, S., Cozzani, E., Gallo, R., Treatment of Rosacea. Annales de Dermatologie et de Venereologie, vol. 138, supplement 3, November 2011, pages S211-S214.

- Yamasaki, K., Kanada, K., Macleod, D., Borkowski, W., Morizane, S., Nakatsuji, T., Cogen, A., Gallo, R., TLR2 Expression Is Increased in Rosacea and Stimulates Enhanced Serine Protease Production by Keratinocytes. Journal of Investigative Dermatology, 2011, 131, pages 688-697.

www.ingramcontent.com/pod-product-compliance
Lightning Source LLC
Chambersburg PA
CBHW070623290526
45790CB00002B/965

* 9 7 8 1 5 0 8 4 6 3 2 8 3 *